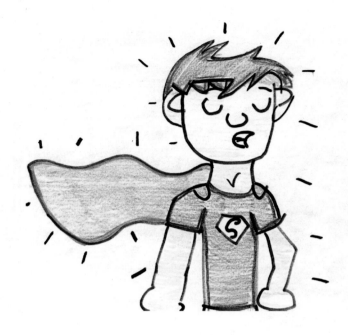

This book is dedicated to all
the Brave Kids visiting
hospitals and doctors.
You are BRAVE.

Special Thank You to our friends Jessica Kahle,
Kendra and Amanda Waltermire and my Yiayia

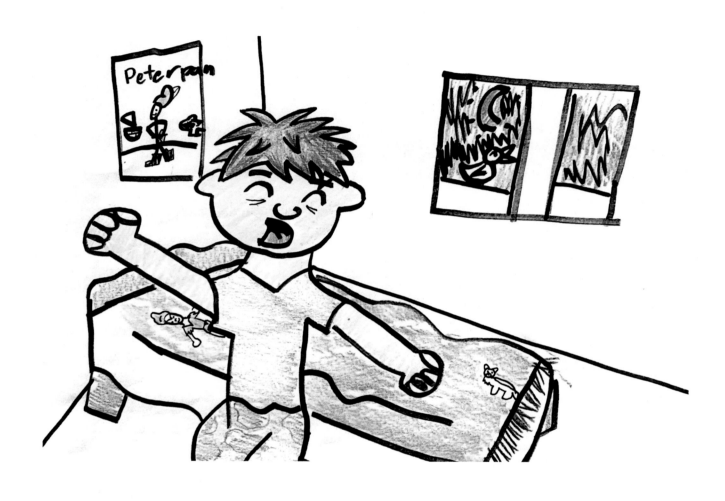

I woke up this morning with the moon. I rubbed my
eyes and stretched my arms.
Today was a different day, and I knew we'd be
leaving very soon.

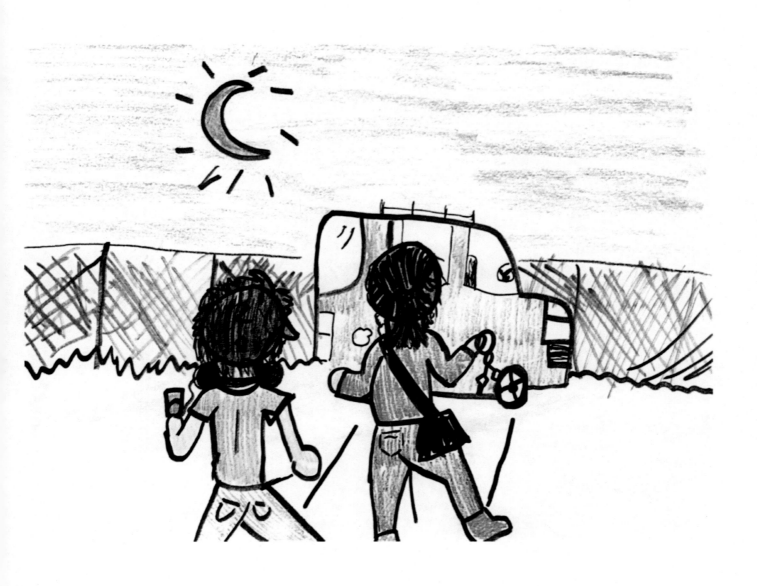

My mom grabs her coffee and keys, and we head out
the door.
I'm tired and not feeling very excited about today.

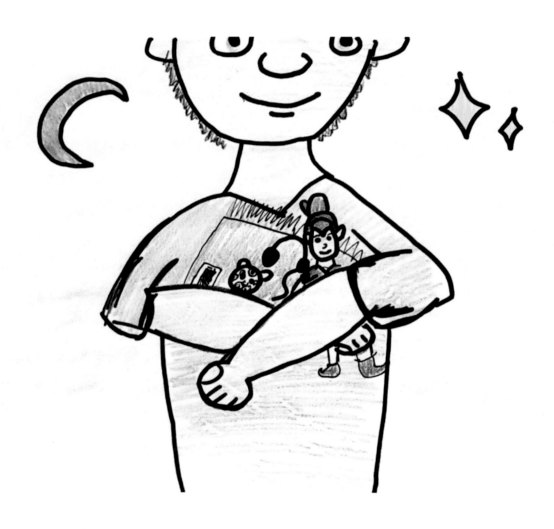

To help me feel better, I bring along some of my favorite things.
I have on my favorite pajamas. I've brought my music and headphones, a few stuffed animals, and my favorite blanket.

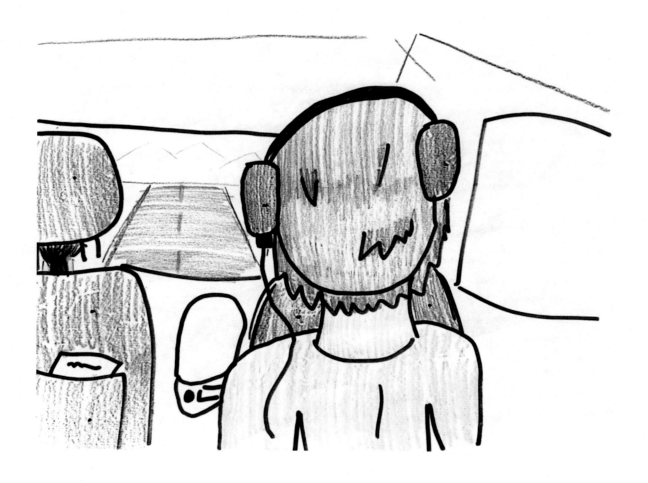

I settle in the backseat of mom's car for the long
drive to San Diego.
Every 3 months, I need to visit a special doctor
called a Hematologist.
A Hematologist is a doctor who studies blood. My
Hematologist is very nice, and I've been seeing her
for 7 years. Each time, she says I am growing taller.

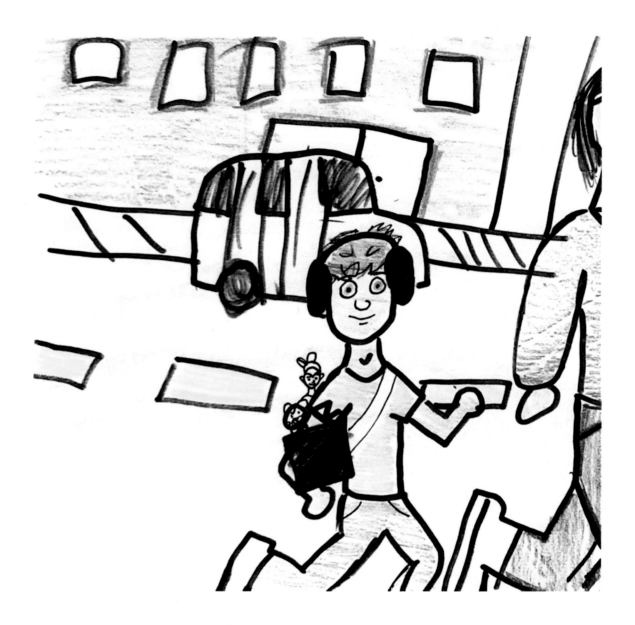

We arrive at the hospital. I grab my favorite things and my mom's hand.

It's still early and my belly growls. I'm hungry.

I am not allowed to eat breakfast on these days. I know after my appointment, mom and I will get a special treat.

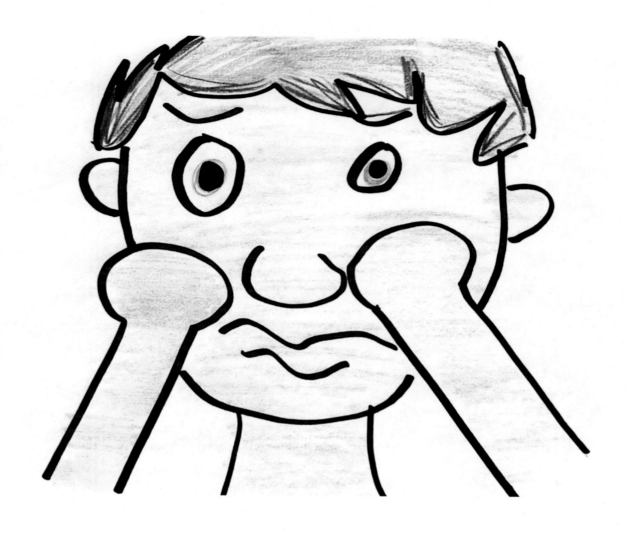

Each time I visit my Hematologist, I have to get a
blood draw. This makes me feel nervous and
worried. I've had blood draws many times before, but
it never gets easy.
I know what I need to do.

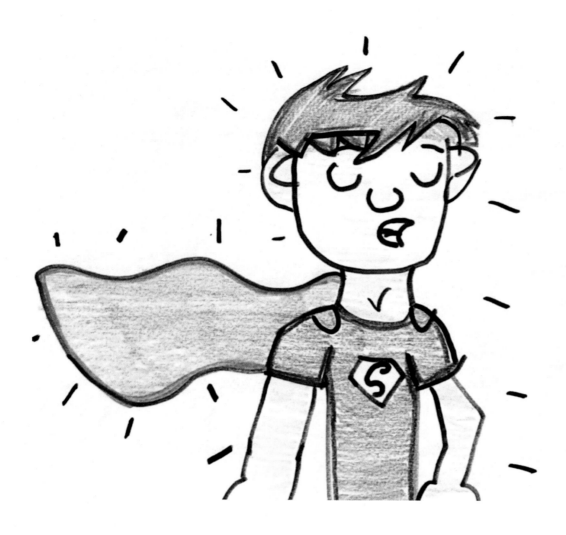

I close my eyes and imagine I am Brave.
Not just any Brave, but SUPER BRAVE.
When you are Super Brave, you feel like you can do anything.
I take deep breaths and remind myself I will be okay.

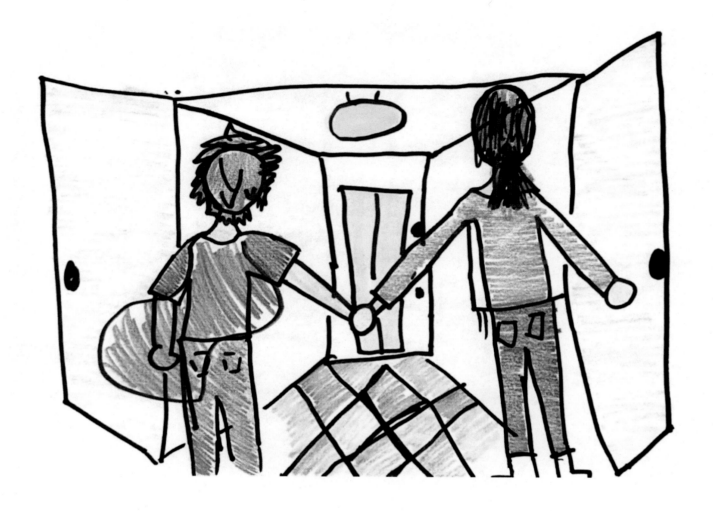

As we walk into the hospital, I begin to feel
Super Brave.
Blood draws are not fun, but I know they are
important.

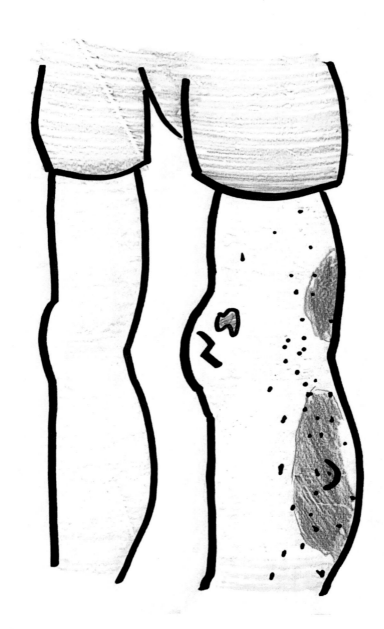

I have Klippel-Trenaunay Syndrome. One of my legs is a little larger than the other with purple birthmarks, called port wine stains, along the side of my leg.

It doesn't hurt, it just looks different than my other leg. My leg has a lot of extra veins pumping blood throughout my body.

Although my leg looks different, I can run, play, and jump like most kids.

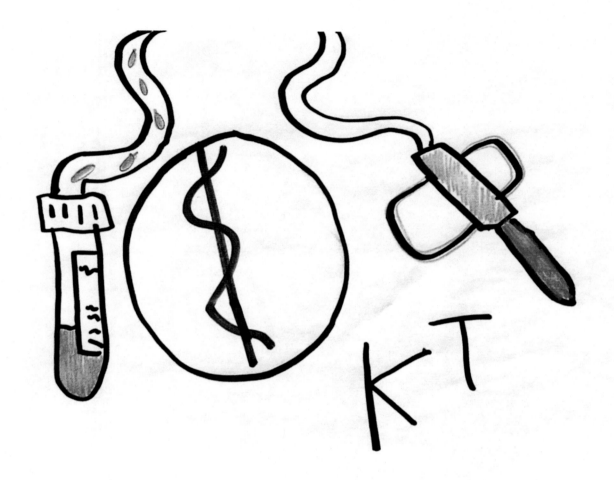

Blood draws are very important for a kid with
KT Syndrome.
When the doctor draws blood from my arm, they can
study the blood under a microscope to make sure I
am healthy. After they take the blood, my body
makes new blood to replace what was taken out.

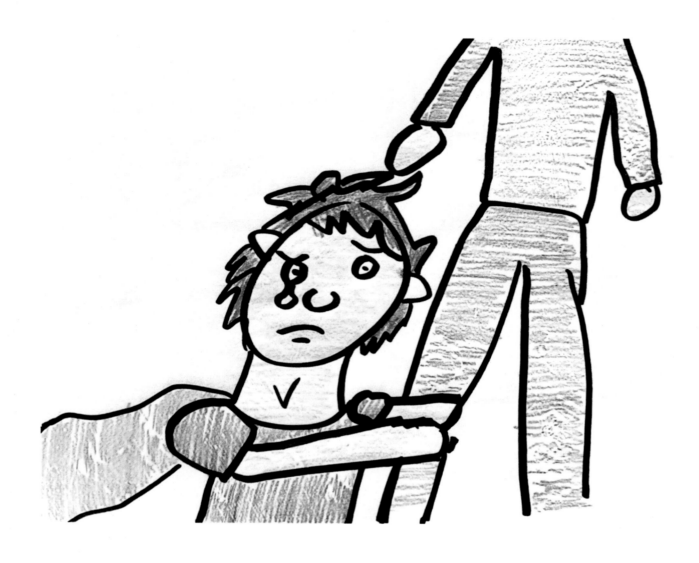

Even with my brave cape, I begin to worry. I know
blood draws are quick, but I also know it hurts a little.
I know I will feel a sharp pain for a second. But once
the needle is in my arm, it doesn't hurt anymore.

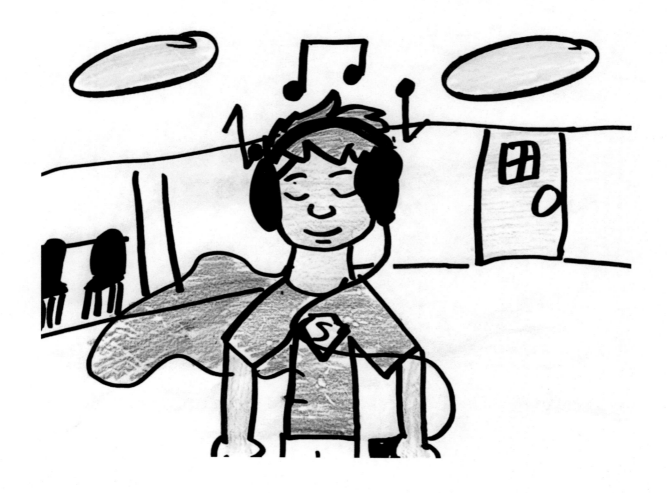

I close my eyes and turn on my favorite music to calm myself down while we wait for the nurse to call me into the room.

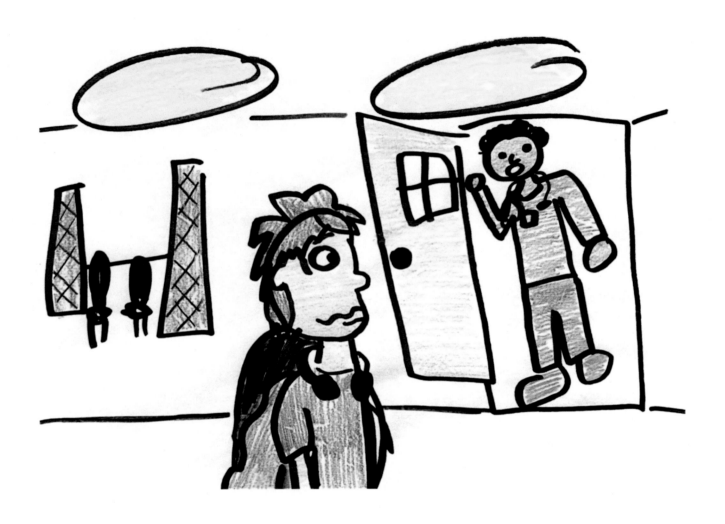

Suddenly, my mom taps my arm and the nurse says
"Jacob" as they scan the waiting room.
It's time to go in.
My brain tells me to run out the door, but I remind
myself that I am Super Brave.

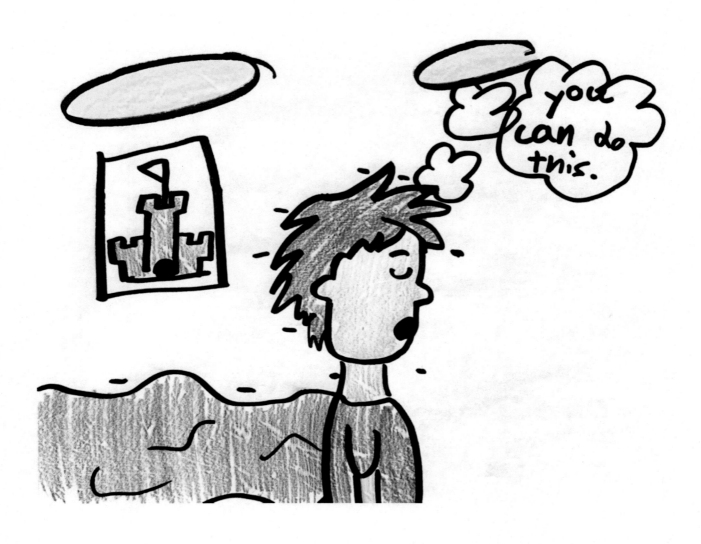

I close my eyes and take deep breaths.
I tell myself, 'You can do this".

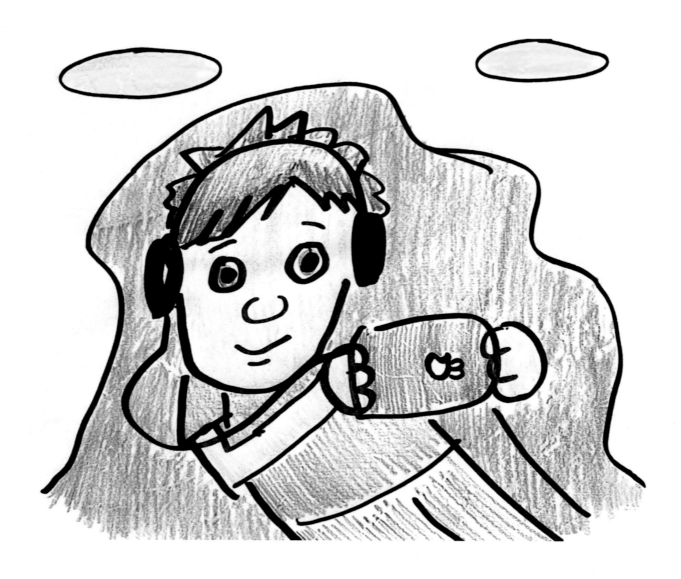

Once inside the room, I settle in with my blanket over my head. While the nurse prepares for my blood draw, I hide out underneath and play my favorite game. My mom talks with the nurse as they check my name on my wristband.

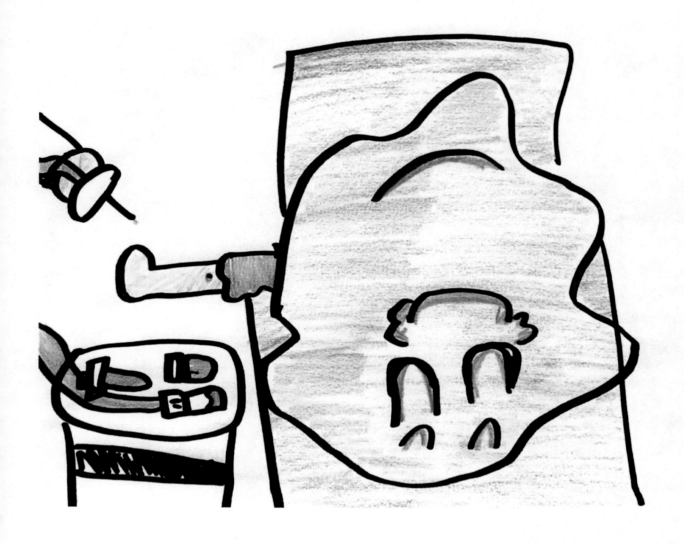

When the nurse is ready, I stick my arm out from
under the blanket. The nurse counts, "1,2,3..."

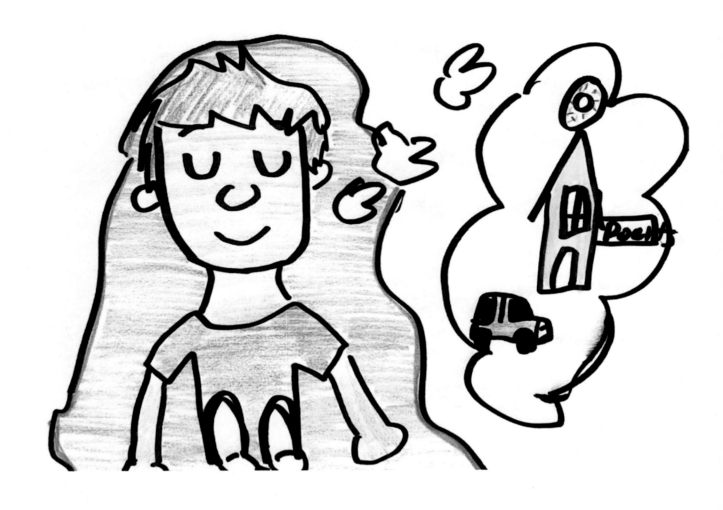

I close my eyes and daydream
of things that make my heart feel happy like:

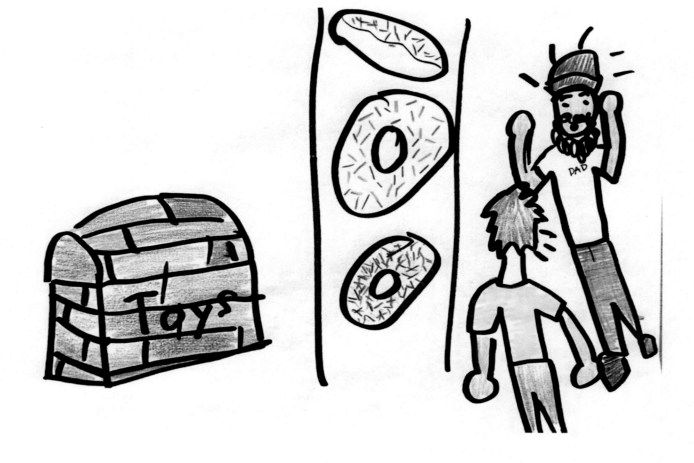

Picking a toy from the treasure box,

eating donuts on the drive home,

and telling Dad, "I did it!'

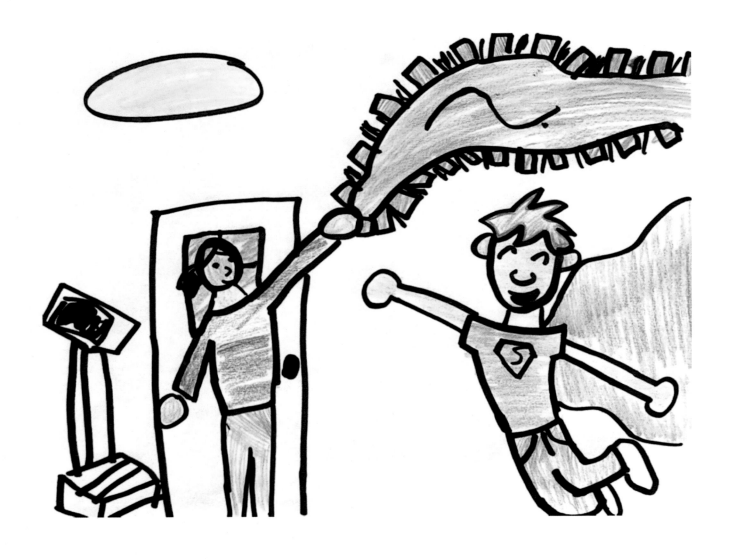

All of a sudden, light shines under my blanket. It's done. I did it!

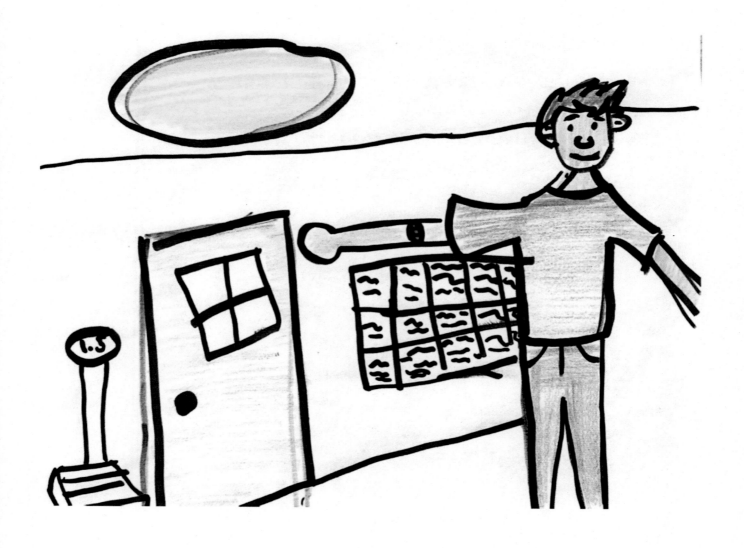

I have a colorful bandaid to cover the spot where the nurse drew the blood. I'm excited to head over to the treasure chest to pick out a prize.

The best part of today was a donut at the
end, with extra sprinkles.
I'm Super Brave Jake and you can be
Super Brave too.

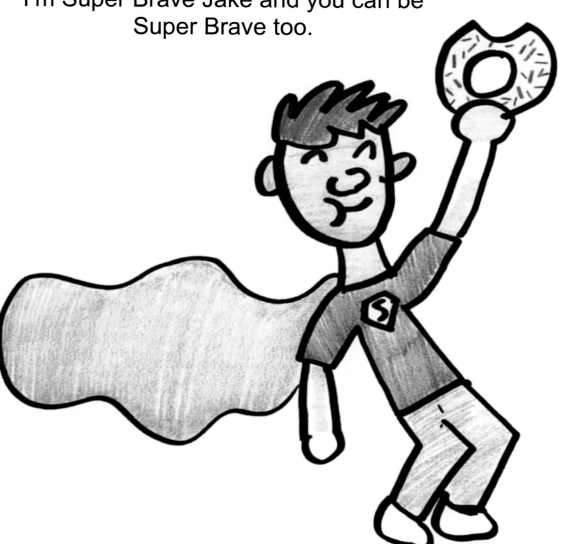

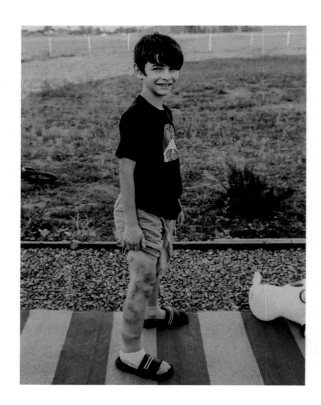
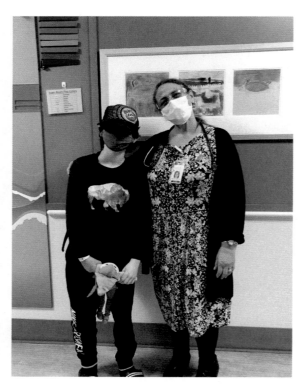

About the Author

Jake Castellano-Meredith is 10 years old. His love of drawing began when he was about 3 he recalls, when he fell in love with Ironman as well as Peter Pan. Besides drawing, Jake loves playing with Legos, building cool forts, riding bikes and playing with his 3 brothers!

Jake wrote Brave Like Jake to "help other kids be more confident and brave when they have to get blood draws or be in the hospital". Jake was born with KTS or Kippel Trenanunay Syndrome, which causes excess vascular and lymphatic malformations to grow. It is different for every person that has KTS but usually involves many hospital visits, blood draws, MRI's, CT scans and sometimes surgery. You can find out more about KT Syndrome by going to
https://www.mayoclinic.org/diseases-conditions/klippel-trenaunay/symptoms-causes/syc-20374152

By Yiayia (Grandma in Greek)

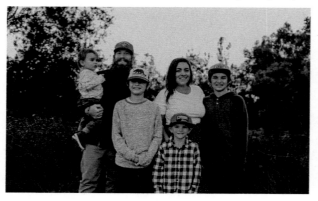
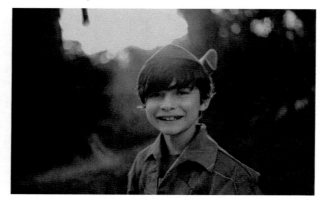

My blood draw tips

By Jake Castellano-Meredith

1. Pick out your favorite clothes. Sometimes, I even wear my pajamas.
2. Gather your favorite items that bring you comfort. I pack them in my backpack to bring along.
3. Stay positive!
4. Talk to your adult about what worries you.
5. Tell the nurse what worries you. They may ask you if you want them to count or just do it. You can choose!
6. You don't have to look. I like to put my head under my blanket, listen to music and squeeze my stuffed animal.
7. When you are done, you may get a treat! My mom will stop for donuts each time. I even bring them home to my brothers.
8. If you can't do it, it's okay. Sometimes, I have to try again, too. Just remember to Be Brave.

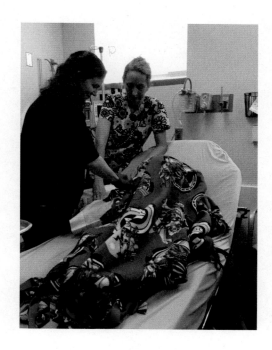

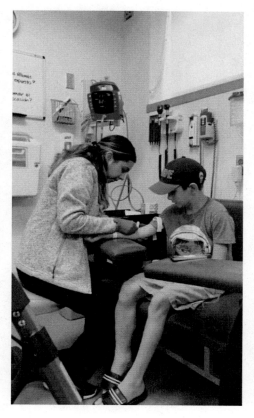

Made in the USA
Monee, IL
03 February 2022

89579402R00017